The Healin

Make Your Own CBD Oil at Home

How to Extract, Use and Heal with Cannabis Medicine

By

Jonathan Seaman

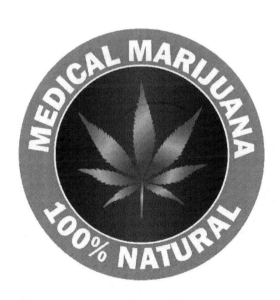

Published by:

www.Valenciapub.com

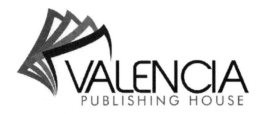

Valencia Publishing House
P.O. Box 548
Wilmer, Alabama 36587

Cover & Interior designed

By

Alex Lockridge

First Edition

Disclaimer:

s meant to provide information about the

alue of Marijuana derived CBD rich Hemp

alth benefits. . The author has made

ʼ ensure that the information in this

ʼ. However, it should be noted that the

growing and the consumption of

ㄱ different countries; hence, readers

ᵉ their own discretion and abide by

untry for growing Marijuana.

t intended to be a substitute for

ʼ doctors. The readers are

hysician in matters relating to

ㄱey start using this herb based

ਰed here are for information

ʼming to cure any diseases

ᵉ suffering to seek proper

CONTENT AT A GLANCE

FOREWORD

I FIRST learned about the medicinal benefits of marijuana through a Dutch friend who was born and raised in the Netherlands where marijuana has been legal for many years now. It was 1994 when I first got interested in learning more about the healing effects of marijuana, but not much data was available back then, as internet was just at its infancy at that time.

As a self-proclaimed Naturopathic healer, my interest just grew over time. Around the end of 1996, when California legalized marijuana for medical use, I was finally able to get more research data on the topic. For some reason, I always had this belief that marijuana holds a big secret under its leaves most of which we just haven't discovered yet.

At first, Marijuana was only used as a painkiller in the medical field as the last resort for terminal patients that were suffering from AIDS, Cancer, and other such deadly illnesses. But after 2005, that started to change in a big way, researchers and doctors started seeing the true medicinal value of marijuana and the healing effects of its various ingredients like THC, CBD and Hemp oil. It was like opening a floodgate, so much started to pour in and so fast that it was truly overwhelming for most researchers.

I too was consumed and overwhelmed with all the information. But I am sure some of you may not know all these details but most of you should remember when Dr. Sanjay Gupta of CNN did a medical breakthrough program of a 5 years old girl in New Jersey that was suffering from an acute case of Epilepsy where she was having 6-10 seizures a day and on modern medicine could stop that.

Long story short, when the parents found out about the new marijuana-derived medical research, they took their daughter and started the new treatment immediately. Only after a few dosages, she started to recover, and from 10 seizures a day she is now down to one or two minor ones maybe once a month! Just imagine the power of Marijuana. Here is a link to an article about Dr. Sanjay Gupta's 'Weed' show.

http://www.drugpolicy.org/blog/little-girl-helps-give-sanjay-gupta-new-perspective-marijuana

I am sure you didn't buy the book to hear me try to prove the benefits and healing power of this amazing plan call marijuana. But I wanted to tell you at least why I wanted to share some of my research and findings as I still believe, there are more amazing discoveries to come in this field, this is just the beginning, and I wanted to share my excitements with you.

My goal in this book is to share some proven facts about marijuana, and by facts, I mean the healing power and actual medicinal value of this plant, nothing more. I share what and how you can find healing through Cannabis derived CBD oil. Now that Cannabis is being legal is many states, it is much easier to find these medicines without going outside the country.

Lastly, before I get started, next time you vote, if you see an option for legalizing marijuana or medical or otherwise, please vote Yes and let's bring healing to everyone in every state, country and eventually in this great world of ours.

INTRODUCTION

BEFORE I get started, I just wanted you to know, even though I have studied, tried and tested many research methods, but this is book is far from those boring data and research outcomes, it is not a research paper either. I originally wrote this book for the people I help in their healing journey. So this should be an easy read for anyone wants to learn what marijuana really is, what's in it, and how they can cure and or heal various diseases.

So, let me start with a little background and then we will break down the plant and what each part does. Sounds good? I promise you it will not be boring.

Marijuana is known by a number of names and has just as many debates surrounding its use. Unfortunately, a good amount of the debates surrounding this plant and its uses is clouded by inaccurate and confusing information (I have found that out the hard way many times).

The medical and psychoactive effects of marijuana are caused by a number of unique chemicals known as cannabinoids. In this book, I'm going to simplify and break down what you need to know about marijuana and its main medical component which is CBD.

Lastly, I as shared some process of how you can extract CBD oil from marijuana, before you try that, please be sure you understand that making your own CBD oil will not work as a medicine simply because the few cannabis derived medicine that are out there have many other ingredients and goes through a process which we cannot duplicate at home. So if you are trying out any of the processes, do it for practice but not with a goal of curing any diseases. As this would be impossible to make such medicine at home.

So let's get started.

WHAT IS IN MARIJUANA?

TO DATE, science has identified 86 cannabinoids in both the natural marijuana plant and chemically synthesized cannabinoids. The main psychoactive ingredient in marijuana is the delta-g-tetrahydrocannabinol, referred to as THC (this is the part that gives people the "high" feeling). Other cannabinoids have either medicinal or psychoactive elements or both. Some of these include Cannabidiol (CBD), Cannabinol (CBN), Cannabavarin (THCV), Cannabigerol (CBG), Cannabichromene (CBC), THC, Cannabicyclol (CBL), Cannabitriol (CBT) and Cannabielsoin; among others. Let's take a moment to consider the four most commonly used cannabinoids.

THC

Since THC is the main psychoactive nature in marijuana, it is often used to measure the herb's potency. The typical concentrations for THC are as follows:

➢ Inactive hemp - Less than 0.5%

- Marijuana leaf - 2 to 3%

- Higher-grade marijuana - 4 to 20%

The highest concentrations of THC are found in seedless buds known as sinsemilla. You can also get high concentrations of THC in extracts, tonics, and hashish or concentrated cannabis resin.

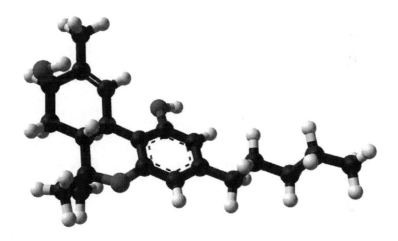

THC doesn't naturally occur in its active form within the cannabis plant. Rather, it occurs in an acidic form known as tetrahydrocannabinolic acid or THC acid (THCA). The THCA is converted to THC when burned in a cigarette or heated in cooking through a heat-propelled reaction called decarboxylation.

Eating raw marijuana won't have any strong psychoactive effects because the THCA is inactive. However, as the plant ages, some THCA undergoes decarboxylation.

I know it sounded boring for me to mention all those long wired names but stay with me and it will get more interesting, I promise.

CBD

This is the second most common cannabinoid and is the most prevalent in hemp varieties of cannabis. CBD lacks any noticeable psychoactive effects and doesn't really interact with the body's cannabinoid receptors. However, there is plenty of evidence that shows CBD has medicinal properties.

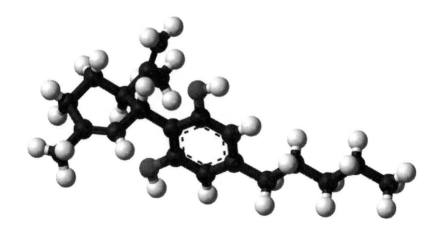

CBD will also work along with THC to augment its medicinal effects while moderating the psychoactive effects. Researchers have also found that CBD has anti-psychotic properties which reduce anxiety and panic reactions associated with THC.

Although CBD can be taken by itself for a number of medicinal benefits that I'll discuss later. However, evidence does show that CBD is biphasic; meaning the effectiveness can be diminished if the dose is either too low or too high.

CBD and THC acid are simultaneously produced. In the marijuana plant, the precursor for both is a cannabinoid called cannabigerolic acid. Each cannabinoid is produced by a different enzyme that acts on the cannabigerolic acid.

This means it is hard to find a plant that has a high level of both CBD and THC. Depending on the breed, some marijuana plants are naturally high on THC while relatively low on CBD and vice versa. People that use marijuana for recreational purpose always look for the type that are high on THC as that is what gives them the pleasure of being a heighten state of mind.

Lately, some of the hydroponic marijuana are gaining popularity for their highly potent THC level.

Hemp plants will often lack the enzyme that produces THC, so CBD is often prevalent. However, most consumer grade marijuana has significantly low levels of CBD since growers selectively breed out the CBD enzyme in favor of producing more THC (since that is people want, and that is where the money is).

CBN

The third most common cannabinoid found in marijuana is CBN. This is basically a byproduct of the chemical breakdown of THC.

CBN lacks both strong medicinal and psychoactive qualities of THC and is often only found in degraded or poorly-preserved marijuana plants.

FLAVONOIDS

In addition to the active ingredients, I listed above, cannabis also contains over 20 flavonoids. Most of these are common in most of plant life, but some called cannaflavins are exclusive to just cannabis.

These flavonoids typically have anti-inflammatory and antioxidant properties.

Marijuana will have different highs and medicinal effects based on the types of cannabis. These variations are there because of different chemical concentrations of cannabinoids and flavonoids in each unique type of marijuana plants.

For the purpose of this book, I am going to look at the main medicinal cannabinoid which is also known as CBD. The first thing I want to do is briefly discuss the interesting history of CBD and marijuana.

HISTORY OF CBD

The first references to cannabis are found about 2,700 years ago in Persia when a spiritual teacher named Zoroaster wrote a sacred text of over 10,000 plants; one of which was hemp. Cannabis extracts were also recommended by Hippocrates, the founder of western medicine.

Cannabis was also tied to Christianity in AD 45, through the Ethiopian Coptic Church. According to this church, the use of marijuana was used as a sacrament descended from a Jewish sect known as the Essenes.

Later in history, Queen Victoria's physician prescribed medicinal cannabis for the Queen's menstrual cramps (I too was surprised when I read this first time). Sir Russell Reynolds went on to write about medical marijuana in the first edition of the British medical journal. Another British doctor of the time, Sir William Osler, used CBD oil for migraines.

During the Revolutionary War, soldiers were often paid with cannabis. Also, farmers were encouraged to grow hemp by George Washington and Thomas Jefferson to make more paper and rope along with clothing and ship sails. The Egyptians had used hemp sails about 3,000 to 4,000 year prior.

There was the mini history lesson, hope I didn't bore you with it too much, but I think it is clear that cannabis has played a major role throughout history.

It has only been recently that there has been a struggle regarding the medical legality of THC and CBD. The most important thing to consider is how each of these ingredients interact with the human body. Let's start by looking at THC.

HOW MARIJUANA WORKS IN OUR BODY

WHEN someone smokes marijuana or ingests it in some other form, THC, and other chemicals are entering the body. The chemicals work their way to the brain through the bloodstream and then distribute throughout the rest of the body. THC is the most powerful chemical in marijuana and is primarily responsible for the "high" that people associate with marijuana.

Marijuana is often smoked since it is the fastest way to get THC and other chemicals into the bloodstream. When the smoke from marijuana is inhaled, it goes directly to the lungs.

The lungs are lined with alveoli or tiny air sacs where gas exchange happens. Since these alveoli's have greater surface area than the skin, it makes it easier for THC and other marijuana compounds to enter the body.

Marijuana can also be eaten where the stomach absorbs the marijuana and finally sends some of the chemicals into the bloodstream. The bloodstream then takes it to the liver and the rest of the body. The stomach takes longer to absorb THC than the lungs. This means that users who eat or consume marijuana by mouth have lower THC levels, but the effects will last longer.

EFFECTS ON THE BRAIN

Once THC enters the bloodstream, it typically reaches the brain within seconds and starts to take effect. Marijuana users typically describe the initial experience as relaxing and mellow. Often colors will be more intense, and other senses become enhanced. Later, some users may feel paranoia and panic. The THC interaction in the brain is what causes these feelings. To understand just how marijuana affects the brain, you need to know more about the parts of the brain that THC effects.

In the brain, the cells that process information are called neurons. The neurons can communicate with each other through chemicals called neurotransmitters. These neurotransmitters fill the gap or synapse between two neurons and bind to protein receptors to allow various functions in the brain and body to being turned on or off as needed.

Neurons have thousands of receptors that are specific to individual neurotransmitters. Foreign chemicals such as THC can mimic or block the actions of neurotransmitters and interfere with these normal functions.

The brain has groups of cannabinoid receptors in several places. These receptors can influence affective activities such as short-term memory, coordination, learning and problem-solving.

These cannabinoid receptors are activated through a neurotransmitter known as anandamide. Like THC, this is a cannabinoid, but one produced by your own body. THC mimics anandamide, which means THC can bind with cannabinoid receptors and activate the neurons in the brain; causing the effects on the mind and body.

The highest concentrations of cannabinoid receptors are found in the hippocampus, cerebellum, and basal ganglia. The hippocampus is located within the temporal lobe and is important for short-term memory. When THC binds with these receptors, it can affect recollection of events. THC can also impact coordination which is controlled by the cerebellum. The basal ganglia works for unconscious muscle movements, which is why marijuana impairs muscle coordination.

WHAT AND HOW CBD WORKS

CBD is the second most common component of the marijuana plant and the main non-psychoactive component (You won't get "high" if you consume this). In recent years, scientists and physicians have become interested in this component. However, it still isn't clear exactly how CBD has a therapeutic impact on the molecular level in the body.

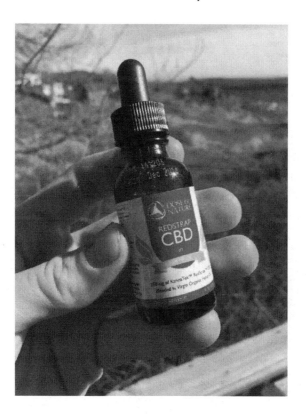

Cannabidiol is known as a pleiotropic drug, meaning it produces many effects through a variety of multiple molecular pathways. CBD acts through receptor-independent channels and binds with a number of different non-cannabinoid receptors and ion channels. There are a few ways CBD provides therapeutic effects and healing to human body.

HOW CBD WORKS IN THE BODY

CBD doesn't make people high because it isn't psychoactive like THC. Within the human body, there is an endocannabinoid system with receptors throughout the brain and body.

THC primarily activates the CB1 and CB2 receptors, while CBD doesn't directly impact these receptors.

CB1 AND CB2 RECEPTORS

The cannabinoid receptors in the human body are responsible for processes like regulation of mood, pain sensation, appetite, and memory.

These receptors are activated by endocannabinoids produced by the human body and plant cannabinoids found in hemp or cannabis. These receptors are grouped into two main categories: CB1 and CB2.

CB1 receptors are typically located within the central nervous system, with smaller amounts found within the liver, kidneys, and lungs. CB2 receptors are found within the immune system and hematopoietic blood cells.

CB1 is involved in the production and release of neurotransmitters; cannabis products (like THC) that have psychoactive effects will stimulate these receptors. CB1 receptors are also involved in the lipogenesis process within the liver and seem to help with the maintenance of homeostasis or the body's internal equilibrium. Studies have suggested that CB1 receptors can also influence pleasure, concentration, appetite, memory and pain tolerance.

On the other hand, CB2 receptors have an impact on the immune system and work with a variety of functions such as immune suppression or programmed cell death. Studies have suggested that these receptors can modulate the pain sensation and could play a role in a variety of diseases from liver and kidney problems to neurodegenerative diseases.

CBD doesn't stimulate these two receptors; rather, it work with other receptors such as vanilloid, adenosine and serotonin receptors. For example, when activating the TRPV-1 receptor Cannabidiol can regulate body temperature, pain perception, and inflammation. CBD inhibits the FAAH enzyme, a compound that activates the CB1 receptor. This minimizes the THC activation of CB1 and reduces the psychoactive effects.

When CBD activates the adenosine receptors, it provides anti-anxiety and anti-inflammatory Cannabidiol effects. The adenosine receptors are involved in releasing dopamine and glutamate. Dopamine impacts cognition, motor control, motivation and reward mechanisms. Glutamate plays a major role in excitatory signals involved in memory, learning, and cognition.

A high concentration of CBD can also activate the 5-HT1A serotonin receptor which has anti-depressant effects. This receptor is involved in processes such as pain perception, appetite, nausea, and anxiety.

Lastly, CBD will block CPR55 signaling. This decreases bone reabsorption and cancer cell proliferation. CPR55 is found through the brain and is linked to the modulation of bone density and blood pressure along with cancer cell proliferation.

As I've stated before, CBD blocks the psychoactive effects of THC. This is why many researchers and doctors combine CBD with THC for treatment purposes. However, you can get positive effects of Cannabidiol without any THC presence.

So you can choose to get the benefits of CBD by buying products made only from the non-psychoactive CBD. Let's consider some of the major benefits you can get from both marijuana and CBD.

HEALTH BENEFITS OF CANNABIS

CURRENTLY, only 6% of medical studies focus on the medicinal properties of marijuana. The following health benefits can be applied to both THC and CBD. However, it is important to note that smoking THC in too large amount for non-medicinal purposes can lead to adverse side effects and some serious complications. It is best to stick with medicinal dosing only to see appropriate health benefits.

health effects of cannabinoids

Cannabis plants can exhibit wide variation in the quantity and type of cannabinoids they produce. The mixture of cannabinoids produced by a plant is known as the plant's cannabinoid profile. Selective breeding has been used to control the genetics of plants and modify the cannabinoid profile.

	THC-A	THC	THC-V	CBN	CBD-A	CBD	CBC-A	CBC	CBG-A	CBG	
Pain Relief	X		X			X		X		X	analgesic
Reduces inflammation	X	X	X		X	X		X			anti-inflammatory
Suppresses appetite			X								anoretic
Stimulates appetite		X									appetite stimulant
Reduces vomiting and nausea		X				X					antiemetic
Reduces contractions in the small intestine						X					intestinal anti prokinetic
Relieves anxiety						X					anxiolytic
Tranquilizing, used to manage psychosis						X					antipsychotic
Reduced seizures and convulsions	X					X					antiepileptic
Suppresses muscle spasms		X				X					antispasmodic
Aides sleep				X							anti-insomnia
Reduces the efficacy of the immune system		X									immunosuppresive
Reduces blood sugar levels						X					anti-diabetic
prevents nervous system degeneration						X					neuroprotective
Treats psoriasis						X					antipsioratic
Reduces risk of artery blockage						X					anti-ischemic
Kills or slows bacteria growth						X		X		X	anti-bacterial
Treats fungal infection						X				X	anti-fungal
Inhibits cell growth in tumours/cancer cells	X	X			X	X		X			anti-proliferative
Promotes bone growth						X					bone stimulant

These statements have not been evaluated by Health Canada, National Health Service or the Food and Drug Administration. Always consult with your physician before taking any medication. Effects of these individual cannabinoids are from peer related scientific literature. Trends in Pharmacological Science, Volume 30, Issue 10, October 2009, P515-527

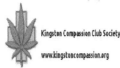

Kingston Compassion Club Society

www.kingstoncompassion.org

As I mentioned before, my work is not advocating the use of marijuana for pleasure or get "high," but it is to see and understand the bigger picture marijuana is showing us. My goal is share the hidden healing effects of this super wonder plant. Let's take a look at some of serious diseases it can heal.

GLAUCOMA

Glaucoma increases pressure in the eyeball which can damage the optic nerve and cause complete loss of vision (my father suffers from glaucoma, I know how serious it is).

Cannabis can be used to treat and prevent eye disease. According to the National Eye Institute studies from the early 1970s have shown that marijuana can lower intraocular pressure in individuals with glaucoma. By slowing the progression of glaucoma, it can prevent blindness.

TOBACCO AND LUNG HEALTH

In January 2012, the Journal of the American Medical Association published a study that shows marijuana doesn't impair lung function and can actually increase lung capacity. Please read it again. Can you imagine that? It is really true!!

EPILEPTIC SEIZURES

A 2003 study showed that marijuana can prevent epileptic seizures. The findings were published by the

Journal of Pharmacology and Experimental Therapeutics. The active ingredients in marijuana control seizures by binding to the brain cells that are responsible for controlling excitability and relaxation.

DRAVET'S SYNDROME

During research for the documentary "Weed," Dr. Gupta found a family that was treating their 5-year-old daughters Dravet's Syndrome, a severe form of seizures, with a medical marijuana strain high in Cannabidiol and low in THC.

I shared the story about CNN's Dr. Sanjay Gupta's Weed program where he showed that five year old girl with a severe case of epileptic seizures. She is the living proof of what this herbal medicine can truly do for human.

CANCER

In 2007, the California Pacific Medical Center in San Francisco reported that CBD may prevent cancer from spreading. Cannabidiol prevents cancer by turning off a gene known as Id-1 according to the study published in the Molecular Cancer Therapeutics.

Cancer cells make more copies of this gene than non-cancerous cells and allows cancer to spread throughout the body. A few studies done in the U.S., Spain and Israel have also suggested that cannabis has the ability to kill cancer cells.

ANXIETY ATTACK

Researchers at Harvard Medical School in 2010, suggested that some of marijuana's benefits can come from reduced anxiety; which improves mood and act as a sedative. For some this can help relieve pain and suppress nausea.

ALZHEIMER'S DISEASE

A study by Kim Janda of the Scripps Research Institute suggests that marijuana may be able to slow the progression of Alzheimer's disease. This study was done in 2006 and published in the Journal of Molecular Pharmaceutics.

The study found that marijuana slows the formulation of amyloid plaques by blocking the enzyme that makes them in the brain. These plaques are responsible for killing brain cells and causing Alzheimer's.

MULTIPLE SCLEROSIS

The Canadian Medical Association Journal published a study that suggested marijuana can ease the painful symptoms of multiple sclerosis. Other studies have also suggested that marijuana can help control muscle spasms.

HEPATITIS C

Hepatitis C treatment comes with some harsh side effects including fatigue, nausea, muscle aches, loss of appetite and depression.

In fact, many aren't able to finish the treatment because of these side effects. However, a study in the European Journal of Gastroenterology and Hepatology in 2006 found that those who used marijuana had less side effects and the treatment effectiveness increased.

INFLAMMATORY BOWEL DISEASE

Those with inflammatory bowel diseases such as Crohn's Diseases and Ulcerative Colitis were covered in a study in 2010 by the University of Nottingham that found chemicals in marijuana interact with the cells in the body that are involved in gut function and immune responses.

Compounds in marijuana can decrease the permeability of the intestines that lets in bacteria.

ARTHRITIS

In 2011, researchers announced that marijuana alleviates pain, reduces inflammation and promotes sleep in order to help those who have rheumatoid arthritis.

WEIGHT LOSS AND METABOLISM

The American Journal of Medicine published a study that suggested marijuana smokers are skinnier than the average person and have a better metabolism. While this isn't true in all cases, those who smoke marijuana often has a healthier response to process sugar in the body.

LUPUS

Medical marijuana is starting to be used to treat autoimmune diseases such as Systemic Lupus Ertyhematosus. Some of the compounds in marijuana have a calming effect on the immune system which can help with the symptoms of Lupus.

PARKINSON'S DISEASE

A recent research done in Israel has shown that marijuana can reduce pain and tremors to improve quality of life for Parkinson's patients. In addition, it showed a marked improvement in fine motor skills for patients as well.

PTSD

In some states, marijuana is already approved for the treatment of PTSD. Natural cannabinoids will help regulate the body systems that cause fear and anxiety.

DIABETES

Studies involving CBD have shown to prevent the development of diabetes in mice. While Cannabidiol doesn't directly affect glucose levels, it does prevent the production of IL-2 by splenocytes. This is important because it helps with many autoimmune diseases.

As you can see from the following table, each compound in marijuana has multiple benefits; but the most come from CBD.

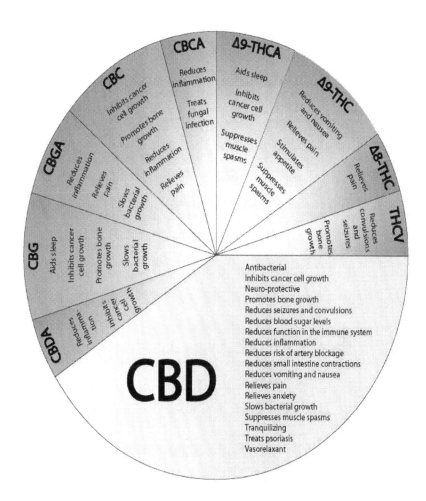

CBCA
Reduces inflammation
Treats fungal infection

CBC
Inhibits cancer cell growth
Promotes bone growth
Reduces inflammation
Relieves pain

CBGA
Reduces inflammation
Relieves pain
Slows bacterial growth

CBG
Aids sleep
Inhibits cancer cell growth
Promotes bone growth
Slows bacterial growth

CBDA
Reduces inflammation
Inhibits cancer cell growth

Δ9-THCA
Aids sleep
Inhibits cancer cell growth
Suppresses muscle spasms

Δ9-THC
Reduces vomiting and nausea
Relieves pain
Stimulates appetite
Suppresses muscle spasms

Δ8-THC
Relieves pain

THCV
Reduces convulsions and seizures
Promotes bone growth

CBD
Antibacterial
Inhibits cancer cell growth
Neuro-protective
Promotes bone growth
Reduces seizures and convulsions
Reduces blood sugar levels
Reduces function in the immune system
Reduces inflammation
Reduces risk of artery blockage
Reduces small intestine contractions
Reduces vomiting and nausea
Relieves pain
Relieves anxiety
Slows bacterial growth
Suppresses muscle spasms
Tranquilizing
Treats psoriasis
Vasorelaxant

CBD OIL EXTRACTION AND PRODUCTION

THE main point of CBD oil is to get a CBD-rich oil high in medicinal benefits. The most effective way to do this is to use high-CBD marijuana plant as the raw ingredient. After you have a good strain of CBD, you need to choose a good manufacturing method.

There are various extraction methods; each with their own pros and cons. Those who want a pure and clean CBD oil are likely to use a different method from a commercial producer. Let's take a look at the various methods of extraction.

CO2 EXTRACTION

This method uses carbon dioxide under high pressure and extremely low temperatures to isolate, preserve and maintain the purity of the CBD medicinal oil. This is often considered the safest method of extraction also purest and the cleanest.

Since this process has highly-controlled aspects, the cannabinoids integrity is always maintained at a higher level. It also removes green chlorophyll to leave a clean-tasting product. However, this method doesn't work well for small-scale producers since it requires expensive equipment and a large learning curve.

Here is an animated YouTube video that shows the whole process, take a look at it:

https://www.youtube.com/watch?v=oJa8dzE0LqE

SOLVENT EXTRACTION

This is the method typically used for small-scale CBD oil production due to its low cost, easily obtained equipment and simple process.

Some typical solvents include butane, grain alcohol, isopropyl alcohol, hexane or ethanol. Some do consider this process dangerous due to the use of highly flammable solvents such as butane and various alcohol. I personally do not recommend using solvents such as butane or pure grain alcohol. As using such highly flammable solvent can destroy some of the therapeutic plant waxes and decrease the medicinal value of the CBD oil. But there is a much safer and truly efficient way you can do this when you follow some simple yet precise procedure. In this process, I use ethanol and not butane or any pure grain alcohol. Once you read the procedure and watch the video, you will know why I say it is simple and easy to follow.

To do this properly, you need the followings:

1 Drip Coffee Maker

Few Coffee filter paper

1 lighter

2 Small glass bowl

1 Large glass bowl

1 large plastic spoon

1 fine strainer

16 oz. bottle of isopropyl alcohol or Ethanol (60% pure)

Bag of Dry Cannabis

1 Home water distiller machine

Process:

Mix dry cannabis with alcohol in a large glass bowl. Mix properly by using a plastic spoon. Let it soak for a few minutes. Then use the strainer to separate the liquid from the solid. Next, put a paper coffee filter inside the coffee maker (don't turn the coffee maker, just let it drip) and pour the liquid so you can separate the fine dust of cannabis from the liquid. Once you have the liquid, use a water distiller to separate the ethanol from the oil.

Once the oil is separated, pour it in a small glass bowl and put it on the coffee pot warmer and turn the coffee maker on so the glass bowl can heat up and let the tiny ethanol particles evaporate. Leave it on there for few hours. The end product should a dark brownish looking thick oily substance that is 100% pure CBD oil.

Just to make sure there is no ethanol left in there, dip a paper clip into the liquid then try to light it with a lighter, if it catches fire then you need to leave it on the coffee pot warmer for few more hours.

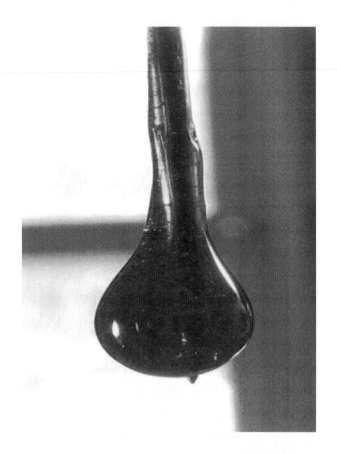

Here is a clear YouTube video of how it is done, take a look

http://tinyurl.com/CBDOIL-Extraction

CARRIER OIL EXTRACTION

A safe and inexpensive option is to use carrier oil to extract CBD oil. Although this method will produce a perishable product that needs to be kept in a cool, dark place. Olive oil is the preferred option since it also provides healthy Omega acids. This option is also only use for CBD oil that is eaten or topically applied and not smoked.

SYNTHETIC VS. WHOLE PLANT FOR CBD OIL

When it comes to making CBD oil, one of the most important things to consider is whether you are going to use synthetic or whole plant CBD. Let's consider which option is best.

Quite simply, a February 2015 article published in the journal Pharmacology and Pharmacy discussed a study from Israel that documented the superior therapeutic properties of whole plant CBD cannabis extract when compared to synthetic, single-molecule Cannabidiol.

The study found that the administration of pure, single-molecule CBD had a bell-shaped dose-response curve. This meant that when the amount of CBD reached a certain point, the therapeutic impact declined greatly. This is a characteristic of all single-molecule CBD that is manifested in bell-shaped dose responses. It poses a serious obstacle that limits the usefulness of CBD oil from a clinical context.

In testing that compared both types of CBD oil, the tests confirmed the findings of preclinical research. A different dose response pattern was observed in whole plant CBD oil.

The whole plant CBD rich oil extract had a direct, dose-dependent inhibition. Also, the testing found that a small amount of whole plant CBD was needed for positive effects while a larger amount of synthetic CBD was needed for the same effects.

So, in a nutshell, it is very clear that if you are looking for clean, potent and natural rich CBD oil, it is best to go with the whole plant and not the synthetic ones.

CHOOSING THE RIGHT CBD THERAPY

There are many forms of CBD therapy available, and you can use it in a variety of ways. The most appropriate method of CBD use is one that provides you with the optimal therapeutic dose for the desired duration with as few side effects as possible. Let's look at the various delivery methods for CBD.

THROUGH SMOKING

Cannabis is often smoked in a joint or pipe. When inhaled the smoke allows compounds like CBD and THC to be absorbed into the lungs and then the bloodstream and lastly to the blood-brain barrier.

The effects of inhaled cannabis often occurs within a few minutes and starts to wear off within two to three hours. Smoking is often used for acute symptoms that need quick resolution. It is easy to titrate a dose by inhalation. However, smoke contains some ingredients that may prove irritating to the lungs.

BY VAPORIZING

Using a vape pen or other device to vaporize marijuana can offer the same immediate effects of smoking. However, a vaporizer heats the cannabis rather than burning it. This means it is a healthier alternative to smoking.

There is a book on how to smoke and consume various cannabis products via electronic cigarettes and vaporizers. You can look for it in most any online book stores. The book title is Weed This Way. By Nathan Farley. I found this book by doing research, and I was surprised as till that day I didn't know marijuana can be used in vaporizer type devices, so I bought the book, and sure enough it was true.

TINCTURES

These herbal remedies are made by dissolving the active ingredients of marijuana in alcohol or other solvents. The effect, duration and dosing of these remedies is similar to those of edibles.

SUBLINGUAL SPRAYS

These are often made from cannabis extracts and may be mixed with other substances such as coconut oil. The concentrate is sprayed under the tongue and absorbed through the oral mucosa.

The initial effects are often felt within five to fifteen minutes. This method is a good option for a consistent, discreet and timely dosing option. You don't need to do any preparation, and you don't have the lingering smell associated with smoking.

EDIBLES

This includes any foods or snacks cooked with cannabis-infused oil, butter or ghee (clarified butter). The effects of this dosing can last between four to six hours, longer than the inhaled option. However, it takes longer for initial dose to start to take effects at about thirty to ninety minutes.

This makes edibles the better option for chronic conditions that need a steady dose throughout the day. The biggest risk in this option is overconsumption, making it more difficult to titrate dosage. It is best to take a small dose and then wait an hour before determining if you need more.

CAPSULES AND GEL CAPS

Cannabis oil can be found in a capsule or gel cap just as you would a vitamin supplement. The effect, duration and dosing of this option is similar to the edible option.

CANNABIS TEAS

Cannabis prepared in an herbal tea form includes a high amount of CBD and THC in the raw "acid" form because the heat for steeping tea is less than the temperature required for decarboxylation that turns CBDA into CBD and THCA into THC.

Since cannabinoid acids don't bind with receptors in the brain, cannabis tea isn't inebriating. Although CBDA and THCA still have therapeutic properties, very little research has been done on these compounds. So, there is not enough supporting data to validate this one way or the other.

VIA JUICING

Raw cannabis juice is similar to teas since it isn't heated. It contains CBDA, THCA, and other non-psychoactive cannabinoids. It is difficult to get precise dosing with this option, but the health benefits are thought to be significant.

TOPICAL AND SALVE APPLICATIONS

Cannabis tinctures and oil can be infused into a balm, lotion or ointment that is directly applied to the skin. These are a good option for pain, inflammation, infections and skin conditions. Since they are applied topically, they don't have any inebriating effects.

CANNABIS OIL EXTRACTS

This option can be taken orally, sublingually or topically. Concentrated cannabis oil extracts can also be used as an ingredient to vaporize or cook. Some cannabis oils have an applicator for measured dosing. These are often very potent. The time of onset and duration of effect will vary based on the method of administration.

WHAT IS THE PROPER CBD DOSAGE

EVEN as medical marijuana and CBD become legal in some states; many doctors are still reluctant to prescribe cannabinoids because they aren't sure of the dosing. CBD Cannabidiol isn't something covered in medical school pharmacology courses.

It has only been in recent years that medical scientists are developing a dosing schedule for medical marijuana, medicinal hemp and all types of extracts such as CBD. CBD rich hemp oil comes in a variety of concentrations and forms.

I do believe in next 5 to 10 years most medical doctors will be trained on the CBD Cannabidiol and will be able to start writing prescription for them as well.

PERSONALIZED DOSING

Cannabis is a very personalized medicine. The specific treatment regimen is based on each person and the condition they are trying to treat. For maximum benefit, some choose a cannabis product that contains both CBD and THC since they interact to enhance the therapeutic effects of each other.

However, a person's sensitivity to THC need to be determined when setting up a ratio and dosage for CBD-rich medicine. Many people can consume a reasonable amount of cannabis without feeling too high or dysphoric.

For others, THC can be quite unpleasant. CBD will help to lessen or neutralize the high effects of THC. This means the greater of the CBD to THC ration, the less of a 'high' you'll get.

The following information I'm going to share is meant to be a guideline and a reference point. Everyone is different and reacts differently to CBD dosing. It is always best to start small and then gradually increase your dose until you get the desired results. The first step to determining effective treatment is to find your ratio.

FINDING THE RIGHT RATIO

Dosed cannabis medicine is available in many forms as we've already discussed above. All of these cannabis medicines have varying ratios of CBD and THC that are specifically calibrated to meet the needs and sensitivities of the individual patient.

Many patients taking cannabis for anxiety, depression, spasms and pediatric seizure disorders find it is best to start with a moderate dose of CBD-dominant remedies such as a CBD:THC ratio of more than 10:1. A low THC remedy, while not intoxicating, isn't often the best therapeutic dose. A combination of CBD and THC often has a greater therapeutic effect and covers a wider range of conditions than CBD or THC alone.

Patients with other conditions such as cancer or neurological diseases often benefit from a balanced ratio of CBD and THC. Research has shown that a CBD:THC 1:1 ratio is most effective for neuropathic pain. Finding the right therapeutic use of cannabis requires a careful, step-by-step process of starting with small doses, observing the results and then gradually increasing the amount of THC.

BIPHASIC EFFECT

All cannabis compounds have a biphasic property. This means that a low and high dose of the same substance will have opposite effects. Small doses of cannabis often stimulates while large doses sedate. While not lethal, too much THC can amplify anxiety and mood disorders.

CBD doesn't have any known adverse side effect at any size dose, but drug interactions can present an issue. Too much CBD could be less effective than a moderate dose.

Always remember when it comes to cannabis therapy, less is more is often the best approach.

8 GUIDELINES FOR DOSING

When it comes to cannabis medicine dosing you often want to follow the same basic steps:

❖ Determine how you want to take cannabis.

❖ Determine your ratio.

❖ Start with a low dose, especially if you are new to cannabis medicine.

- ❖ Take a few small doses throughout the day rather than one large dose.

- ❖ Use the same dose and ratio for a few days and observe the effects before adjusting if necessary.

- ❖ Don't overdo it.

- ❖ Be aware of potential side effects. In addition to amplifying anxiety and mood disorders; other possible side effects are dry mouth, dizziness, and faintness.

- ❖ Talk with a health professional. This is especially important if you have a history of alcohol or drug abuse, mental illness or are pregnant or breastfeeding (talk a doctor before you get started).

HOW MUCH SHOULD YOU TAKE

For cancer patients to increase appetite - 2.5mg of THC with or without 1mg of CBD for six weeks.

For chronic pain - 2.5-20mg CBD for an average of 25 days.

For epilepsy - 200-300mg of CBD for up to 4 and 1/2 months.

For movement problems such as Huntington's Disease - 10mg per kg of CBD for six weeks.

For sleep disorders - 40-160mg CBD.

For multiple sclerosis - 2.5-120mg of a THC-CBD combination for 2-15 weeks.

For schizophrenia - 40-1,280mg CBD for up to four weeks.

For glaucoma - a single dose of 20-40mg CBD.

However, you also need to make sure you are getting the best type of CBD oil. Consider the following when purchasing your CBD oil.

BUYING CBD OIL

OFTEN if you want to buy CBD products, you need to do a little work to find accurate information. While CBD is increasing in popularity, the internet is typically filled with false information. Also, CBD is still a misunderstood dietary substance. It is often confused with THC, the psychoactive ingredient in cannabis.

Contrary to these popular misconceptions, CBD is actually legal worldwide and is very safe to use. There are no psychoactive elements to CBD and no risk of getting high.

Once you are ready to try CBD products, you need to consider several factors such as brand, CBD concentration, type of product and your individual needs. So let's take a look at what you need to know.

BUYING CRITERIA

CBD comes in a variety of shapes, sizes and forms. You need to know how to compare similar products and distinguish nearly identical products to make an informed decision when buying CBD. Let's consider three important criteria in buying CBD.

VOLUME

For many people, an important buying criteria is how much CBD the product contains. Obviously, each product is going to contain a different amount of CBD, and it is important to know how much you are ingesting. When determining volume, make sure it is specifically CBD and not just the overall hemp oil.

HEMP OIL

CBD is typically measured in two volumes: CBD as we've already discussed and hemp oil. The hemp oil volume refers to the total volume of hemp oil within a product. While hemp oil has its own therapeutic benefit, when buying CBD products you want to be specifically considering the amount of CBD in a product.

A good way to explain this is with the example of fish oil. Fish oil supplements often contain a specific amount of total fish oil and a specific amount of DHA and EPA; the important substances in the supplement.

So when you are looking for fish oil supplements you want to look at the total DHA and EPA quantities per pill and not the total fish oil. The same applies when purchasing CBD as well. Look at the specific amount of CBD rather than the hemp oil volume.

CONCENTRATION

Concentration is another important characteristic of a CBD product. Concentration refers to the abundance of CBD compared to the total volume of the product. The concentration you choose will depend on how much CBD you want to take and what product you choose to get it from.

It is recommended that new users take 1 to 2 mg daily at first. Depending on your metabolism, body weight, and desired affects you may choose to start with 3 mg, and you can always increase the size as your body becomes accustomed to it.

When used consistently, CBD has maximum efficiency just like a daily multivitamin supplement.

This is because it takes your body awhile to adjust to the chemical compounds in CBD. Since there are no psychoactive or dangerous components to CBD, you can easily increase your dose to find the right concentration for your individual needs.

10 THINGS TO LOOK FOR WHEN CHOOSING CANNABIS MEDICINE

When choosing a cannabis medicine there are a few things you need to look for:

- ❖ CBD-Rich Products - Choose once that include both CBD and THC.

- ❖ Clear Labels - Look for labels that clearly show the quantity and ration of CBD and THC per dose, a manufacturing date and a batch number of quality control.

- ❖ Lab Testing - The best products are tested for consistency so you can be sure they are verified free of mold, bacteria, pesticides, solvent residues and other containments.

- ❖ Quality Ingredients - You should choose products that only include quality ingredients. Avoid anything with corn syrup, GMOs, Trans fats or artificial additives.

❖ Safe Extraction Methods - Avoid any products that are extracted with toxic solvents such as BHO, propane, hexane or other hydrocarbons. Solvent residues can be dangerous, especially for immune-compromised patients.

❖ Cannabis vs. Industrial Hemp - Hemp is often lower in cannabinoid content when compared to whole plant cannabis. A large amount of help is needed to extract a small amount of CBD, increasing the risk of contaminants drawn from the soil. Whole plant cannabis will also enhance the therapeutic benefits.

3 TRAPS TO AVOID

As more people are turning to CBD products for medicinal benefits, the market for hemp-derived products has dramatically improved. The increase in popularity has led to an increase in misleading marketing and deceptive advertising.

There are three main tactics that non-reputable companies will use to try and get you to buy their CBD oil. Consider the following three traps to avoid when buying CBD oil.

QUALITY VS. PRICE

With so many CBD products on the market and individual desperate for relief from sometimes painful symptoms, it is easily to simply buy the cheapest CBD oil you can find.

However, cheaper doesn't always equal quality product. When you search for CBD oil, you will get over five million results online. The majority of these producers and distributors don't offer proof to support their product claims.

While lower prices make products more attractive, you do well to consider quality over price.

To make sure you are getting a safe and effective product you want to consider quality and not price.

When it comes to CBD, quality is defined by the higher concentration of Cannabidiol since this means more powerful effects and a better investment of your money.

EXAGGERATED PRODUCT CLAIMS

By reading this book, you are already taking a step to avoiding this trap. You want to know about the real properties and benefits of cannabinoids before you try to buy them. Hemp oil and CBD oil are two different products as we've already discussed. And neither of them are same as medical marijuana.

You'll find many CBD products that claim they can cure different conditions such as cancer or you'll read how the hemp oil has miraculously healed patients from a variety of conditions. It is best to avoid products that sound too good to be true. CBD oil is a powerful product, but it isn't a cure all for sure, but so far we know that it does have an amazing healing power.

ENSURE IT IS NON-PSYCHOACTIVE

Some hemp and marijuana products on the market have psychoactive compounds. However, CBD is scientifically proven to be non-psychoactive. This makes it important to check the label before you buy CBD products and only choose those that are low in or free of THC.

If you are worried about getting high from marijuana products, then you want to stick with ones that only contain non-psychoactive products. Again, be aware of products that seem too cheap. Making good CBD oil requires expensive technology.

When you carefully choose your CBD oil and avoid commonly found dishonest marketing campaigns, you will be able to get a quality product that is sure to provide the therapeutic affects you are looking for. However, one thing many people are still concerned about is the legality of CBD oil. This is a very difficult and gray area.

CBD AND FEDERAL LAW

WITHIN the cannabis universe, there are two types of plants that are very broadly categorized: hemp and drug plants. Hemp plants include any plant grown for fiber or seed oil. Drug plants include THC-rich euphoric plants and non-euphoric CBD-rich plants. The difference in these two plants is the resin content. Most hemp plants are low resin, and drug plants are high resin.

Industrial hemp is often a low resin agricultural crop that is grown from pedigree seeds. They are usually grown as a cluster of one hundred tall, skinny plants per square meter and then harvested by machine and manufactured into a number of products.

Drug plants are a high resin horticultural crop that is often grown from asexually reproduced clones at one to two plants per square meter. They are hand harvested, dried, trimmed and cured.

RESIN LAWS

At one time, federal law defined marijuana based on its resin content. In the 1970 Controlled Substances Act, resin was mentioned three times within the definition of marijuana.

The law basically stated that while certain parts of the plant such as the mature stalk and sterilized seed are exempt from the legal definition of marijuana; flowers, leaves, and stick resin wherever it is found on the plant are not exempt.

Federal law is clear on the point that the resin from any part of the marijuana plant or any preparation made from the resin is not allowed under law. Fiber produced from hemp stalk and oil pressed from hemp seed are legally okay, but the resin isn't. Little confusing? Well, read on.

When it comes to the medicinal and recreational use of cannabis, the resin is the most used portion. The resin contains both THC and CBD, along with a number of other components like I discussed at the start of this book.

The resin is found within the heads of tiny, mushroom-shaped trichomes on the female flowers or buds. To a lesser extent some resin can be found on the leaves.

THE THC ISSUE

It is clear that since the beginning, the Federal government assumed resin content was the main factor in separating marijuana from industrial hemp. However, federal law has changed to include a caveat that officially characterizes industrial hemp as nothing containing more than 0.3% THC by dry weight. This small amount of THC won't have any euphoric effect.

This figure comes from a 1976 taxonomic report by Canadian scientists Ernest Small and Arthur Cronquist. The 0.3% figure was never meant to be used as legal definition, but it eventually did. The Drug Enforcement Administration started everything by trying to ban hemp food products, including hempseed oil.

On October 9, 2001, the DEA published an "Interpretative Rule." This stated that any product, containing any amount of THC is classified as a

Schedule 1 controlled substance. This effort fell apart due to the actions of the Hemp Industries Association (HIA). In February 2004 the HIA won when the Ninth Circuit Court of Appeals rejected the ban on hemp food based on substantive grounds.

However, this court decision didn't affect the legal status of CBD. The Controlled Substances Act remained as the law.

Although CBD hemp oil purveyors often cited the February 2004 ruling as a basis for claiming, their products are legal in all states. The court decision never mentioned CBD, and many maintain that the ruling didn't legalize CBD.

THE FARM BILL

The 2004 court decision also didn't mention anything about a THC percentage. It wasn't until ten years later when the Federal Farm Bill was passed. Also known as the Agricultural Act of 2014, this is when the 0.3% THC rule was added to the federal law.

Section 7606 of the Agricultural Act included the definition for industrial hemp for the first time in US history and provided a clear distinction from marijuana. Cannabis was classified as hemp, not marijuana, as long as no part of the plant exceeded the 0.3% concentration of THC.

Section 7606 of the Farm Bill didn't mention resin, which also created a legal exception for growing industrial hemp in the United States under state-approved pilot research programs. This loophole opened opportunities for industrial hemp advocates.

For the first time in many years, American farmers could cultivate industrial hemp on domestic soil on a provisional basis rather than rely on hemp grown products from abroad that could be marketed in the United States. However, it was limited to states that legalized industrial hemp farming. Growing industrial hemp outside of state-sanctioned pilot research is still not allowed by federal law.

KENTUCKY CBD MOVEMENT

The first state to start a multifaceted federally approved pilot program to study farming fiber hemp and hemp for seed oil along with farming CBD-rich plants for medicinal oil extraction was Kentucky.

Under state and federal law, it is currently legal for certain licensed individuals in Kentucky to breed, cultivate and harvest industrial hemp, formulate products and ship them across state lines; this includes CBD-rich oil concentrates.

Since Kentucky chose to follow federal sanctioned agricultural programs, local hemp farmers could gain access to certified, pedigree seed stock from European and Canadian sources after getting a DEA Controlled Substances Import and Export Permit.

This pedigree seed supply is vital in maintaining the uniformity and consistency of a large-scale, machine-harvested hemp crop. Today, there are hundreds of cultivars who can meet global demands for hemp products. -*0

However, industrial hemp plants aren't optimal for getting CBD-rich oil. So Kentucky farmers starting look for high-resin, CBD-rich drug plants from state sources where cannabis is legal for therapeutic use.

THE COLORADO MOVEMENT

Colorado's state industrial hemp program is also growing a number of high-CBD/low-THC cannabis.

However, much of Colorado's start up hemp industry isn't compliant with Section 7606 of the Agricultural Act of 2014. Rather than growing hemp for research purposes according to federally sanctioned pilot initiatives, Colorado bypassed protocol and moved straight into a large-scale commercial cultivation.

While it is legal to grow industrial hemp, make hemp products and distribute these products within Colorado, federal law prohibits them from being transported across the border and the sale of hemp oil products. Although CBD isn't legal in all 50 states, hemp oil is. Several Colorado startup companies are marking CBD-rich hemp oil to sell in all 50 states.

There are a few farmers in Colorado who are actually growing a high-resin, CBD-rich drug plant and defining it as hemp. These growers often harvest the crop several weeks before maturity and when the resin content reaches its peak.

This allows them to keep the THC level at 0.3% or less. However, this isn't always the case. Whether any plant measures slightly above or below the 0.3% THC limit won't affect the quality of the CBD-rich oil extract and its therapeutic benefits.

REVISITING INDUSTRIAL HEMP

The new peaked interest in the medicinal potential of CBD has been responsible for the increased popularity of industrial hemp growing in the United States.

The resurgence of the industrial hemp market in the United States is a step forward both economically and ecologically. However, it also points to ongoing problems when it comes to cannabis legality and prohibition.

CBD has been responsible for loosening federal law when it comes to industrial hemp. However, federal law still currently prohibits American farmers from growing any high-resin CBD-rich drug plant that even remotely exceeds the 0.3% THC limit.

Despite the fact that these high-resin cannabis plants are better for getting CBD-rich oil than a low-resin industrial hemp plant. Cannabis oil needs to be safely extracted without toxic solvents, and it needs to be made into high quality products that don't contain artificial ingredients, chemical preservatives, thinning agents or corn syrup.

If the goal is to have a large CBD-rich oil yield, then it doesn't make sense to decide whether a plant is qualified as a source of CBD simply based on the THC content. The best source of CBD-rich oil is a whole plant that is high-resin, CBD-rich; no matter how minor the variation of THC is present in that plant.

Today, CBD oil is actually a co-product or byproduct of industrial hemp grown by farmers from around the world for other purposes. If farmers sell their unused hemp biomass to a business that can extract CBD from leftovers they can make some additional money.

This practice is common among large-scale hemp growers in Canada. However, this practice is technically illegal, unregulated and it often filled with pesticides and is extracted using toxic solvents.

THE ISSUE OF HEMP OIL

When grown outdoors in test soil that is carefully processed, industrial hemp can be a great source of CBD. However, there are several reasons why it still isn't an optimal source of CBD-rich oil. Industrial hemp often contains less Cannabidiol than high-resin, CBD-rich cannabis.

This means it requires a large amount of hemp foliage to get just a small amount of CBD. This increases the risk of contaminants since hemp is a bio-accumulator, meaning it draws toxins from the soil. This isn't great for making ingestible medicinal oil concentrates.

CBD paste that is derived from industrial hemp and heavily refined is a poor starter material for CBD-rich oil products. Both imported paste and products infused with pure hemp-derived CBD powder found everywhere online often include thinning agents.

For medical patients using a vape pen, it means the oil contains propylene glycol (PG). When overheated, this chemical produces formaldehyde, a known carcinogen. But if the liquid is mixed with vegetable glycerin (VG) then it is safe to vape

If a pure CBD derived product is heavily processed, then it can lack the full spectrum of aromatic terpenes and other cannabinoids typically found in high-resin drug plants.

These compounds work along with CBD and THC to increase therapeutic effects. Whole plant CBD-rich cannabis oil has been shown through scientific research to have a broader range of therapeutic attributes and greater efficacy than single-molecule CBD.

Under current federal law, any CBD-rich plant that has over 0.3% THC is considered marijuana and can't be grown or used for extracting. However, the federal government is more lenient when you are discussing pharmaceutical THC.

Single-molecule THC is a Schedule III drug that you can get through a prescription in all 50 states, even though it has a large psychoactive effect. Schedule III is reserved for therapeutic substances that have a low abuse potential. Whole plant cannabis, on the other hand, is still classified as a Schedule I drug with no medical value.

WHAT THE FDA THINKS

The FDA issued a warning on February 4, 2016, to eight CBD hemp oil retailers. These warning letters were for making unproven medical claims on 22 different hemp-derived CBD products. The FDA also tested for CBD content and found some didn't even contain Cannabidiol. This was the second time the

FDA had sent warning letters to CBD hemp oil businesses for mislabeling products.

Exposing this fraud is important and a good thing for the FDA to do. However, the FDA has undermined its credibility by following the drug war mandate. For example, the FDA issued an advisory memo against medical marijuana on April 20, 2006; which stated that cannabis was both dangerous and not beneficial medically.

Under current regulations, a product can be marketed as medicine unless the FDA deems it safe and effective for specific conditions. However, FDA approval doesn't always mean a product is safe or effective. Studies are routinely falsified by hiding clinical trial data about side effects and negative results. The FDA also often fails to deal harshly with corporate criminals.

CBD ONLY LAWS

The 0.3% THC legal limit is impractical when it comes to CBD-rich oil products. It has become the key factor in cannabis prohibition, and it blocks medical research and patient access to therapeutic options.

So far, 23 US states have enacted their own medical marijuana laws, and 17 states have even passed CBD only laws that allow the therapeutic use of high CBD/low THC products.

None of the CBD only states, other than Kentucky, are complying with federal law when It comes to industrial hemp. There is no clear consensus when it comes to the proper THC limit in industrial hemp. For example, in North Carolina, it is 0.9% while Texas is at 0.5%. Each state government sets their own rules.

Some states have limits on the sources of CBD-rich products and specify a narrow set of medical conditions for which it can be used; while other states don't have these restrictions.

Advocates of CBD only laws argue that it is a step forward in the process for full legalization of medical marijuana. However, there hasn't been any advances in this area in states that have already passed CBD only laws. Most patients don't actually benefit from CBD only laws. Patients require access to a wide spectrum of whole plant cannabis treatments, not just products that are low in THC.

Enough of this legal battle. If you are interested in the legality of CBD products, check with your local law enforcement. Let's move on to taking a look at what CBD users have to say about the benefits they gain from using this therapeutic drug.

REAL TESTIMONIALS

"**A**BOUT 20 years ago, I was diagnosed with a condition called Systemic Mastocytosis. This is a disorder that results in excessive mutation of mast cells throughout the body. Mast cells in a healthy, normal person help to protect from disease and help with healing wounds. When you have my condition, an excess of these mast cells build up in different parts of the body.

Allergens or injury can trigger these mast cells and cause them to release substances that overwhelm the body and cause symptoms such as facial flushing, itching, rapid heartbeat, abdominal cramps, lightheadedness or even a loss of consciousness. Since my diagnosis, I've tried many drugs and treatments. While some would give me a bit of relief, I never was really able to control my symptoms.

I like to spend time outdoors, but encountering pollen would trigger my symptoms; almost to the point of having to stay indoors. I started that CBD about 60 days ago and have never had a recurrence of my symptoms since." - Richard T.

This is just one example of an individual with a difficult condition that is seeing relief though the use of CBD. The internet is full of these testimonials. Let's look at a few more.

Consider just a few of the reviews found on this website:

https://healthyhempoil.com/cbd-hemp-oil-reviews/

"After ten years of regular seizure activity and an anxiety disorder which developed in response to the fear of the seizures, I have been offered a gift of a substance in CBD drops which have reduced the number of seizures and helped ease the anxiety. It has only been a week that I have been taking this wonderful tincture, but my life has changed for the better. I had begun to give up hope. There was a valuable lesson for me. Never give up." - Jessica M.

"It seems to be good on muscle relaxation... I have less spasms on CBD than I did with other meds." - Will T.

"I use this for my Fibromyalgia pains. It works great & I noticed my sleep is very sound. I will not use any traditional pain management meds. It is also safe & effective for my 15 year old dogs hips. Amazing results for her in much smaller doses needed. Thanks, Brandon." - Mark. B.

"I live a very active lifestyle; I run, hike jog whatever I can to get outdoors. But in recent years I had a huge pain in my hips when exercising. I tried so many things to help, but then I tried CBD oil. Now I can hike, run jog and even ride horse pain free!! It also reduces stress. HIGHLY recommended!" - Yolanda L.

Consider the reviews on another website:

https://www.cbd.org/patients-of-care-by-design/patient-testimonials-care-by-design

"Care by Design is the only medication that has relieved my seizures in 27 years. It's helped symptoms of slurred speech, body tremors, cognitive issues and helps keep my muscles relaxed."

"I take Care by Design for pain, arthritis, depression, anger management. Sleep is extremely important to me since I have violent nightmares. Care by Design has helped greatly."

"Hormone injections did not make any difference. After only using CBD-rich cannabis for six months did my prostate has normalize."

"I was diagnosed with mesothelioma stage 3 this year with prognosis of 6 months to live. Your CBD products have helped me manage unbelievably devastating news and physical deterioration.

I've always treated my body with respect, with a good diet, exercise, and vitamins. Now it feels like the rug was pulled out from under me. I'm thankful I have the option of using CBD products to help me deal with severe agitation, sleeplessness, depression, mood swings, and pain. Thank you!"

However, it isn't just the testimonials of people who take CBD that you should consider. Let's see what some doctors have to say about CBD and its therapeutic effects.

WHAT THE DOCTORS SAY

PERHAPS the most famous example of a doctor promoting CBD is Dr. Sanjay Gupta; neurosurgeon and medical adviser. Gupta narrated a "Special Report" on CNN that provided examples of cannabis providing medical benefits.

In the show, entitled "Weed," Gupta interviewed over a dozen people. In the beginning, he visited young parents Matt and Paige Figi who had a five-year-old daughter named Charlotte (about whom I spoke earlier) who suffered from Dravet Syndrome or a severe form of epilepsy.

The parents are straight, never used marijuana and live near Fort Carson. The Figi's recounted their experience with Charlotte and how all conventional treatments weren't working. She was having hundreds of seizures a day, and the doctors were actually considering putting her into a coma to save her life. The father research CBD treatment and now give an under-the-tongue application to Charlotte.

She has begun recovering with seizures down to once a week.

Another doctor to consider the Bonni Goldstein who is the medical director at Canna-Centers. This is a group of medical practices throughout California that educate people about the use of cannabis therapy.

Dr. Goldstein treats children with intractable epilepsy that isn't responding to available treatments. In addition, she also sees a lot of children with autism. She starting to see children with cancer and severe psychiatric disease that hasn't been helped by current conventional medications.

Dr. Goldstein reports that some of the children with intractable epilepsy come to her with developmental delay and other significant problems such as pulmonary problems, GI problems, and immune function problems.

These are children who can't live a normal life and can't attend school. After giving these children CBD oil, many report a decrease in frequency, severity, and duration of seizures.

Another example of CBD use comes from Greg Gerdeman, an assistant professor of Biology at Eckerd

College in St. Petersburg, Florida. He spoke at the Annual Meeting of the Congress of Clinical Rheumatology. In his speech, he was quoted as saying, "Using cannabis or other sources of cannabinoids for rheumatic diseases shows a lot of preclinical promise because of the importance of the endocannabinoid system in regulating inflammation and the adaptive immune response."

Lastly, consider the findings of Dr. Dustin Sulak; the found and director of Integr8 Health. This is a network of holistic health clinics that specialize in cannabis therapies with offices in Massachusetts and Maine. His clinics conducted a study of patients taking opioids.

The study showed that 39% stopped using opioids completely after starting cannabis; 73% sustained the reduction of opioids for over a year, and 39% reduced their dose but were continuing opioids use. These same patients reported that 47% had a reduction in pain greater than 40%. 80% of patients reported improved function and 87% reported an improvement in quality of life.

In addition to individual doctors, you should also consider some major studies and the results that they have shown in CBD use.

The 26th annual conference of the International Cannabinoid Research Society (ICRS) was attended by 297 delegates from 24 countries. The four-day science symposium featured several reports that showed the potential therapeutic applications of CBD. Consider some of these report findings:

Brain Trauma - Spanish scientists reported that when CBD was administered after a stroke in animals, it reduced brain damage, restored neuro-behavioral performance and prevented excitotoxicty from serotonin and dopamine release.

CBD Protection - When hypothermia is combined with CBD it is more effective at protecting the brain function of newborn mammals after a hypoxia-ischemia event.

Neuropathic Pain - Researchers are Temple University determined that CBD and THC work together when treating neuropathic pain after spinal cord injuries.

Cancer - Italian scientists reported that CBD-rich cannabis extract reduced the viability of white blood cancer cells and induced cell death in multiple myeloma cell lines; potentiating the chemotherapeutic effects for prostate cancer.

CBD for Kids - Douglas Smith with Medicinal Genomics discussed the genetic factors that influenced the efficacy of CBD in seizure disorders in children.

GABA Receptors - Australian researchers determined that one of the ways CBD imparts an anti-anxiety effect is by enhancing the GABA receptor transmission. GABA receptors are directly activated by anti-epileptic drugs.

Lower Blood Pressure - Polish scientists showed the CBD can relax pulmonary and enteric arteries in animals with hypertension.

It is pretty clear from both testimonials and doctors that CBD offer therapeutic benefits.

CONCLUSION

WE'VE discussed a lot of information and given you a lot of points of view. It is important to remember that THC (Tetrahydrocannabinol) and CBD (Cannabidiol) are both cannabinoids that naturally occur within the resin of the marijuana plant. Both of these substances interact with cannabinoid receptors within the human body, but the effects of these compounds are vastly different. This is why CBD is looked to for more therapeutic options than THC.

THC

THC is the main psychoactive component fund in marijuana. It is the primary agent responsible for the high feeling associated with those who smoke marijuana. It works by imitating the effects of anandamide, a neurotransmitter that is naturally produced by the body to modulate sleeping along with the perception of pain. THC causes the following:

✓ Relaxation

✓ Altered senses to sight, smell and hearing

✓ Fatigue

✓ Hunger

✓ Reduced aggression

Research studies have shown that THC can help treat the following:

➢ Side effects of chemotherapy by reducing nausea and vomiting while improving appetite.

➢ Multiple sclerosis by improving spasticity and bladder function while reducing painful spasms and overall pain.

➢ Glaucoma by reducing pressure inside the eye.

➢ AIDS by alleviating the symptoms and stimulating appetite.

➢ Spinal injury by lessening tremors.

CBD

CBD has the same chemical formula as that of THC, but the atoms are arranged slightly differently. This variance allows CBD to lack the psychoactive effect of

THC. CBD makes up 40% of cannabis extract, and it provides a strong example of therapeutic effects. CBD causes the following:

✓ Reducing psychotic symptoms

✓ Reducing convulsions and nausea

✓ Reduced anxiety

✓ Reduced inflammation

Research studies have shown that CBD can help treat the following:

➢ Schizophrenia by reducing psychotic symptoms.

➢ Social anxiety disorder by decreasing anxiety.

➢ Depression by reducing symptoms.

➢ Side effects of cancer treatments by decreasing pain and nausea while stimulating the appetite.

THC is classified as an illegal drug. CBD lacks the harmful cognitive effects of THC use. The lower health risks associated with CBD along with its efficacy make it, the better choice for therapeutic applications.

MY LAST WORDS

I HOPE I was able to shed some light into what the medicinal value and healing effects of CBD oil, as that has been my passion for many years now. Often the laws are the ones that can adversely affect research and development of such products, but good news is the laws are changing though at a slower pace, but hey at least they are changing right?

In this last election, we all know few more states just joined others as they legalized medical marijuana. It is a step towards the right direction, let's hope in the next election we can legalize more states, and in few years, all 50 states will follow the same path.

Lastly, I wanted to thank you for buying by book, I know my writing style is not the best, but to my defense, I am not what you may call a real author, nor I am a writer, but I am a researcher. But I assure you the material I shared here are true and authentic.

If you think I added some value in this book, I would love to see a review from you wherever you bought this book from. It will mean the world to me.

For any reason, if you need to get in touch with me, you can email me at: ValenciaPublishing@gmail.com

Thank you, wish you a very happy and healthy life my friends!

65598330R00053

Made in the USA
Lexington, KY
17 July 2017